The poems in Jeanne Bryner's *Smoke* reveal her to be an angel of mercy not only in her work with patients but also in her ability to create poems that comfort and guide us as we face universal fears: sickness, personal and societal abuse, family tragedy, physical pain and emotional longing. Bryner intertwines striking images and perfect metaphors in poems that use nursing as a lens through which to view the world of healthcare as well as the lives of families, communities, and the art of writing. Because she has witnessed moments only a nurse might, she is able to plunge through the poem's surface event to reach the ineffable. Her poems dig deep, reaching what Emily Dickinson called "the zero at the bone."

These poems are not only startling and emotionally engulfing, they are handsome and well built; there are few poets writing today who can construct images and metaphors that are as fresh and as spot on. Joy and tenderness rise in this collection along with anger and forgiveness, but no cloying sentimentality. Bryner takes on birth and death without bypassing either the gruesome or the transcendent. She portrays nursing as an essential human occupation, replete with smells and sounds and fear, and more than once she puts a doctor in his place.

In *Smoke*, Bryner reveals how and why things might go wrong in the hospital, in the home, in the family, in the community—and yet she brings us, always, to the conclusion that what matters is how we care for one another no matter the storm...that we stand by. Her poems reassure us that through such loving care we will be saved.

-Cortney Davis

Also by Jeanne Bryner

Poetry

Breathless
Saquaro
Not Far From Town
Blind Horse: Poems
Tenderly Lift Me: Nurses Honored, Celebrated and Remembered
No Matter How Many Windows

Fiction

Eclipse: Stories   o
The Wedding of Miss Meredith Mouse

Play

Foxglove Canyon

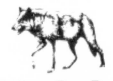

Bottom Dog Press

8-22-12

For Dan,
An amazing
artist & friend.
A loaf of
bread for
the journey!
Love,
Jeanne

SMOKE

Poems

~~Jeanne Bryner~~

Jeanne Bryner

Working Lives Series
Bottom Dog Press
Huron, Ohio

Bottom Dog Press
PO Box 425
Huron, Ohio 44839
http://smithdocs.net

Credits:
General Editor: Larry Smith
Cover Design: Susanna Sharp-Schwacke
Cover Art: Judy Waid
Author Photos: Tammy Streets

Acknowledgments

Sincere appreciation to the editors of the journals and anthologies in which these poems first appeared, some of them in slightly different forms:
Appalachian Heritage: "Afternoon Shift, 1979"
Cancer Poetry Project: Poems by Cancer Patients and Those Who Love Them (Minneapolis: Fairview Press, 2001): "I Will Breathe and Breathe"
Hektoen International: A Journal of Medical Humanities: "When a Friend Asks Me What It's Like to See Someone Die"
Labor: "Silence Gives Consent"
Manna: "Aunt Clara"
Mediphors: "What Nurses Know"
West Branch: "Strawberries"
What's Become of Eden: Poems of Family at Century's End (New York: Slapering Hol Press, 1994): "Where God Lives"
The following poems from *Journal of Emergency Medicine*, by permission from Elsevier Science: "Cotton," 14.2 (1996), copyright © 1996; "Violets," 13.1 (1995), copyright © 1995; "Birch Canoe" and "Rain" 20.3 (June 1994), copyright © 1994; "Saturday Night Emergency Room Conversation," 20.2 (April 1994).

[Additional Acknowledgments on page 93]

Contents

For Sara, Mary Kay, Nancy, David and Ben

Only now can I begin to tell
in how many dreams they've wandered, in how many crowds
I dragged them from underneath the wheels,
in how many deathbeds they moaned with me at their side.

-Wislawa Szymborska
"Memory Finally"

When you pass through the water, I will be with you;
in the rivers you shall not drown.
When you walk through fire, you shall not be burned;
the flames shall not consume you.

-Isaiah 43:2

Bed Bath

Into the morning's sacred space
our backs bend like saplings
in the wind: the nurse
to her washcloth,
the surgeon to his scalpel.

For it is one of the holiest acts
to set a steamy pan of water
upon the over bed table,
to dip and dip your cloth's
whiteness and rotate the soap.

Disrobing the bodies
of the sick, adjusting limbs
and blankets, spreading arms
like wings, both people bow
their heads and become naked.

The hands need no
instruction, for here
palms make a path of swirls
like a wolf circling high grass
to shape her birthing cot.

The small talk of water's
splash is ancient, ancient
also are the brown spots
under each breast, the halo
of hair 'round genitals.

Let us remember our boats
await us; luminous cells
and salts ignite as fire
only to burn out
in blue basins, rest as hazy
light over a distant marsh.

I

I never spoke—unless addressed—
And then, 'twas brief and low—
I could not bear to live—aloud—
The Racket shamed me so—

Emily Dickinson (486)

Strawberries

Sometimes, walking for hours through my shift,
I don't feel the old man's weight on the gurney.
I don't hear the endless rotation of dirty black wheels
against this floor. I don't know how many pulses

I've taken at the end of the week.
The god of water comes to me, calls me,
and I'm a small girl running under a garden hose,
my braids glistening in its spray.

I want to say don't bother me, my Mama
has sent me to pick strawberries, fetch the cream,
and yellow cake is baking in our kitchen.
A man appears in the doorway clutching his chest,

his heart's a maple gray and twisted in a storm;
his breath becomes handfuls of raspy leaves.
A boy now, he gathers them, hands them to his mother.
I go to him, the way I'd just go to anything pale

and shaking, the preacher's wife fainty in her pew.
I hand him my art, two gloved hands, tired feet,
my simple row of needles.
Today, I want brown bouquets

to be the geese returning year after year.
I want it all to go on dancing,
tall grass sweet and hidden
in the marsh, every single wild strawberry.

Leaving the World Behind to Become a Nurse

polish your stethoscope with alcohol, clean it like a blackboard, sit for report next to the coatroom, do all the math twice. in oceans of paperwork, swing your lantern toward voices adrift, close both eyes as you listen to breath sounds and pinpoint the dull lobe with percussion, open wide, say Aaah or Aaha with your mind every minute, every shift. become a pupil in the body's one room schoolhouse. when your inner eye divides the abdomen into four rooms so you can eavesdrop on the gut's pipe fitters, raise your hand. maybe your finger will point to a broken connection, a leaky valve. without diving, marvel at gray pearls hidden in both ears. imagine you are the barking dog beneath a pile of ribs, cold chain wrapped around you, your water bowl upside down. the truck driver with all those tattoos? he's a boy's folded note saying *Please see me. I am here. I am right here.* read edema's Daily Press and the blink of cap refill as your mother's smile, hold on to the capsized boat and throw a rope at the same time, spell pneumonia and nystagmus correctly, try not to melt when it's your turn in the hot seat, learn the difference between a mouth blowing smoke and an idea that's pure fire, don't be a floater. bring waders; nursing's a busy river, your feet must master slippery logs.

Nurse at the Trauma Conference

I'm scheduled to read after the medical examiner,
just before lunch. Where I am now, it's a lucky spot,
after sandwiches and cookies, the crowd
gets sleepy; they work 12-24 hour shifts.

Firemen, paramedics, nurses and docs.
The medical examiner's saying please,
you must be more careful with evidence,
more mindful of what gets tossed or saved.

Someone, he says, threw panties away
(it was a rape). In his sweater vest and bow tie
he might be an aging professor just off sabbatical.
He's telling us how long he's been on the job,

how many parents still practice
the fine art of child abuse, how before he ties
his apron, puts on his gloves,
brings his saw from its place on the wall, he prays

to the god of bones, the god of secrets.
He bends close to those babies and children,
curls his crooked pinky to theirs.
Show me what they did, he says,

I will tell your story.
I will try to make it right.

Witness Trees

These old sycamore trees stand along Baltimore Street in Gettysburg. These trees withstood three days of fighting in and around the small town.

-Report, National Parks Service

I am a tree. A sycamore.
A girl who felt alone
in the field of battle.
Growing up, I was raised

by winds. Hailstorms,
lightning strikes, words
like bullets, blood all over
the ground. Being a tree

there's no protection,
no legs to run away.
Up close, I've seen the
wounded heaped in piles.

Children, women, men.
Cries haunt my nights.
I had to stand and take
the weather, recording pain

circle by circle. Notches
cover my heart, freezing rain
splitting limbs. Some days,
I wished to be blind.

The place you're from?
The people you've loved?
Never leave them behind.
I grew up and grew old.

How bullets missed me
is the story I will my body
to tell. I am a tree,
a sycamore who is still afraid.

Even now, writing this letter,
I tremble. Inside,
I cannot stop shaking.

Bread and Wine:
Poem for My Brothers

There was a swing set in the backyard, children
in the house holding each other like driftwood in sand.
There was never a trial, no arrests or handcuffs, but
our stepmother was a snake, and her venom
reshaped us into a platoon of servant puppets.

We grew quiet, we never sang. Neighbors
who lived near our brown house with green trim
thought of their own shoulders and hurts.
Men rode the buck and tremble of the steel mill's hide,
women felt children's foreheads, washed and hung
winter diapers until their poor hands bled.

On the seven hundred block of the projects
for five summers my brothers, ages four and six,
were prisoners in the bedroom. Yes. Summer prisoners.
They grew pale as candles, heads shaved, little stick arms
fell from their shirts like Dachau's children.

In the eight-by-ten foot space where they slept
a woman who married our father kept them.
Remember Europe's ghettos? How children invent
a New World, a better place? My brothers folded
a spelling book lengthwise and called it a *bat,*

a pair of cotton socks turned inside out became a *ball.*
David pitched. Ben would bat. Soft as mice in rafters
they ran for any noise meant the belt,
going to bed without supper. Monopoly's a lie,
all those GET OUT OF JAIL FREE cards,
better to play marbles, swallow pennies hoping to choke.

Neighbors heard my brothers' voices call through July's
screens like bedsheet ropes dropping from a dormitory fire.
Women taught bedtime prayers, saw the moon's light switch on,
off, counted T-shirts, underwear, blue jeans on our line.
Our neighbors ate meatloaf, cabbage rolls, read gray newspapers,

slept at night. Once or twice, women offered to call
Children's Services, but what house welcomes five faces?
What tent this desert?

Silence is a cell without windows;
for its dirt floor, I have saved all these spoons.
I saw my baby brothers live the life of spiders,
lie wingless as flies upon their beds.

And I will call their names *Bread* and *Wine*.
With a shepherd's staff will I lead them to a fine meadow,
and I will speak of it now and in the time to come.

Aunt Clara

That year my Mama was crying depressed and put away
for the hundredth time, our Daddy drove clear to Fairmont,
West Virginia, to fetch Aunt Clara, my papaw's baby sister.

She was harmless crazy as a honeybee drunk on moonshine
and loved the scent of baby powder. She carried my brothers
straddled on her hips and white puffs trailed her

like dust behind a tractor. We ate tomato soup for weeks
and watched her clean our medicine cabinet with a toothbrush
dipped in Comet. She wore pearly Cat-eye glasses and red

gingham housedresses. Her hair hung short and dark
around her face like shoelaces. She slept on our green couch
with all her clothes on. It was July, and when she took a bath,

none of us could go pee. One Thursday, she called her friend
Sadie Marcus at the Weston State Mental Hospital, talked
two hours about *The Guiding Light* and *General Hospital.*

My Mama got some better and came home rested, quiet.
Two weeks after Aunt Clara left for Fairmont, Daddy
got a letter saying she'd forgot her lower denture, left

it floating in a cup, inside the medicine cabinet she'd cleaned
every single day. By then, Mama was sick again, Daddy didn't
care a spit about Aunt Clara's teeth. Neighbor women, Martha

Jane and Myrtle Louise, tended to us. We ate navy beans and
scared Tammy Rae's baby brother with Aunt Clara's yellowed teeth.
Years later, Aunt Clara died in a mental hospital, her lower lip sunk.

Where God Lives

It is hard to believe in God, even now,
He was always somewhere else. Maybe fishing.
And sometimes I get mad. Like when my sister
was eight and I was six. Daddy went drinking,
left us all alone with my baby brothers.
We were potty-training the chubby one, Ben.

I went to pull him off his potty seat
and his weenie got caught in a crack
of blue plastic. Blood spurted as if I'd chopped
a hen's neck. My sister ran. All four of us crying
now, and me holding Ben's poor wiener
like a bloody worm in a washcloth.

I begged God to stop the warm ooze soaking
through to my palm and held Ben
who yelped louder than Sam the day
we shut his tail in a closet. *I'm sorry,*
please God, help us. I chanted my prayer,
the way you do when you see the train's face
frothing in the tracks, its yellow eyes and teeth
hissing the dark and your car's stalled,
all the doors locked tight.

Our screen door whined, slammed
when my sister brought the women
in their gingham blouses. They found Vaseline
in our cupboards, rocked Ben until he slept,
gave us orange popsicles, threw
the potty seat in the trash.

It is difficult to believe in God, even now,
but I want to say, that day, when I was six
and holding what was left of my brother's dick
in my right hand, God's hair was in pin curls
under a red bandana. He had two names:
Elsie and Janet May. He lived on our street:
the four hundred block of the projects.
He was home. It was August and too hot for trout.

Night

You are twelve years old, early autumn, a day so warm windows, doors stand open. It's Saturday, one sister washing dishes, brothers in their bedroom, your father, step-mother passed out on their bed. Home brew. Whiskey. Today, their tanks already full. Your older sister's pulling brush curlers from her silky hair, teasing it, combing it, lots of spray. Girls meeting tonight, Lori's house. Your sister's president of Y-teens. You need tennis shoes for gym, maybe someone will call you to baby-sit. Money is good. Your father wakes, a grizzly poked by a stick. On his way past your brothers, he crushes a lightbulb with his bare hand. Because it's there. Because he can. When he demands to know who didn't empty the mop bucket, your sister sticks her head out of the bath-room, *Me*, she says. Her hair's done up and her striped louse pressed, it hangs loose over her jeans. You don't know why he grabs her hair and starts punching her face with his fist over and over, why your stepmother decides to join in the bear's dance of punch and choke. Why does a kid keep watching such a scary movie, but there's no afghan to put over your head. And anyway, you think the neighbors have called for help, the cavalry's coming. Snot's running down your face holding hands with tears and from the kitchen your sister says, *They're gonna kill her.* She says it like *we have to do something or else.* What would that be? You have to pee, but the bathroom's too close to those awful sounds coming from your sister's lavender bedroom, those wrenching cries of hurt and hate. When the angels come, at last, and your sister staggers down the hallway bleeding from both ears and her left eye (you didn't know an eye could bleed), an eye swollen nearly inside out, you *feel it* and wince. Her breast's the size of a purple melon, choke marks like rope burns circle her neck. A dirty wet bath towel gets thrown over your sister's face. *Clean yourself up*, your stepmother snaps. In a living room chair, you are an earthquake, you are the epicenter and the needle on the seismograph. So much blood you think your sister will probably die. You cannot speak. Maybe you nod your head, start to lift your hands toward the towel sliding off what's left of your sister's face. No, you cannot. The small animal of your body has crawled into its cave to wait for mercy, to paint what has happened on the walls.

How I Came to Poetry

My seventh grade English teacher stands
in front of the blackboard and taps
her pointer against her palm.
It's no accident our hands are folded, prayerful.

She hates the Beatles, and one day even pulled
her thin hair down to her nose, played
a pretend guitar screaming *Yeah, Yeah, Yeah*
wanting us to learn proper placement of commas.

I'm in the row under the clock, where once she saw me
peek at its face. *Time passes,* she said, *will you?*
Today she's pulled another question from her iron kettle.
When you grow up, what do you want to be?

And when Henry Johns says fireman, someone laughs
in the second row (a Negro fireman?). The undertaker's
kids says lawyer (he's such a brown noser), and of course,
Lucy softly says a mom. Finally, she calls on me, a doctor

or nurse, I say. Her knuckles blanch, she sighs.
To be a doctor, you have to be really smart.
Henry Johns throws me a gap-toothed grin,
a ladder to get us safely out,

me and this little wren I been carrying in my chest.

Goodness

Dear Dr. Wong, Today, I saw our neighbor girl kicking a stroller and smoking. The baby inside was hers. She's not in school on this fine April day. It made me think of my best friend in 1963. Sixteen. Pregnant. I hope you did not get cancer, as I have put off writing this note forever. You probably don't remember my friend's chocolate hair and sad brown eyes, her not-so straight teeth, how she spoke with her face bowed. In her sixth month, her lower jaw locked. Her face was a pale bridge where a car teetered ready to fall. She couldn't talk. She started to cry. I carried warm washcloths, held them to her face. Nothing worked. Her folks weren't home. I bit my lip, ran for the neighbors. They eyed her like she was a dog hit and bleeding in the street. They looked at me. I was fourteen; finally an angel stepped up, drove her to the hospital. Doctors had the good sense to send her to a children's hospital. Two lives were at stake. Lab work, x-rays, lots of searching for any break in her skin. Her belly growing ripe as a melon, its flower blooming inside. First chance, she put her clothes on over her gown, ran into the night. Her sister caught her in the parking lot. No plan, her life all jammed up; she'd never seen lights of center stage. Three days later, Dad took me to visit. I felt she might not be saved. A girl who can't drink or eat? Open mouth drooling, hanging like a wrecked car. By afternoon, her jaw chewed macaroni cheese, a burger on a soft white bun. *How'd they fix you?* I asked. She wiped ketchup from her lip. Some lady doctor, she said, Dr.Wong came to see me this morning, before dawn, sat here on my bed (she patted the sheet). For a long time, she talked to me. Dr. Wong said this here (my friend rubbed her Buddha belly) is a baby, not a sin.

Young Nurse's Lullaby

Your pediatric mentors say, *You'll learn to translate*
toddlers', teens', babies' cries
sounds children make for hunger, pain, distrust, loneliness.
From those four countries, you are a refugee, but the war,
muddy crawl under childhood's fence, making it out,
remain cloudy; no eyes can see those scars.
Working full-time, midnight you lift babies to your hip,
cradle them near your breast, push pink medicine, their IV poles,
humming, always humming. Holding toddlers in your lap
mask and mist of breathing treatments, the old tune drifts
through the room, fixing fresh blankets for croup tents,
your colleagues wonder: this nurse, her strange lullaby.
They watch you from the back streets of their eyes.
You are not the nurse opening complaint's umbrella,
you do not enter morning's report shaking off grumbles
like raindrops. No, you're the new nurse humming
from one room to the other, a melody that's contagious,
how to explain the lullaby's your Mother's voice calling
you home in the dark, some stars already out and you
don't know the Big Dipper's handle from a tricycle,
but you're learning, and your Mom, she's always talking
so fast. Maybe she knows there will not be enough time
to tell it all, to say how it was to hold you close,
how happy she was to teach you one violet song.
Aaah, sweet voices of little people, watering flowers
and humming, apron over your dress,
the best life of your life.

II

There is a defining moment which comes early in a poet's life.
A moment full of danger. It happens at the very edge of becoming
a poet, when behind there is nothing but the mute terrain where,
until then, a life has been lived and felt without finding its formalization.

-Eavan Boland
"In Search of a Language"

Cotton

For Dr. Robert L. Stauter

January in emergency. A girl baby on the gurney.
Terrycloth sleepers, stiff with dried spit up,
and her mother, a denim globe, pregnant again,
says, *Fever, fever all night long.*

Through our too-big gown, I slide infant fists,
thinking how I love babies, every color like balloons,
they smell of talcum and hope, smile at strangers
wearing white coats and masks. The doctor:

Why the cotton in her ears? The mother, *Roaches.*
My five-year-old got one in her ear so I . . .
Me? A nurse, who pulls the fluff away: cotton, cotton.
He sees puckered canals, angry stuff filling each drum.

Eyes closed, he listens, stethoscope moves shiny as
a quarter on the sidewalk of her small chest.
Deep inside he hears: a wino wheezing on a park bench,
a pot of potato soup bubbling over on the hot plate.

Eyes open. *Sounds like pneumonia, we'll get blood work,*
an x-ray. She'll be admitted. I'll be back.
He's Iowa corn, a silk tie under blue, blue eyes.
This mother never believes men who say they'll return.

It all happened years ago, when I was a young nurse.
And now my grandchildren say I'm mixed up—
no wino ever slept in a baby's chest,
and how could roaches nest in a child's ear? —

I was going to say this is a story about
holding back sharp twigs with cotton balls,
how we are happy for what we do not know,
the way you felt before you read this.

Saturday Night Emergency Room Conversation

Sharon called off for afternoons.
Don't get up without help.
This will be tight, another ambulance, room 4.
Were you knocked out?

Our baby won't eat.
My aunt's purse, heart pills.
No, I'm not pregnant.
Was that stuff my baby? Call my Mom,

she's at work. Tell me the name
of this place. *Take a deep breath, hold it.*
We're down a nurse, we need leathers.
Start drinking. My veins are crummy.

This board's killing me. Her brother
shut the door on her fingers, all of them.
Take this mask off of me, can't breathe.
Hi, want to come in for four hours?

Who's the president? He took off. Page
security, page the sup. Apply pressure.
I said, one stick. This baby's mine.
We've been here 6 hours. I only smoke cigars.

The room's spinning. Don't move it, don't touch it.
Can you work a double? Big pinch. Don't move.
Swallow, just swallow. When did you eat last?
First lunch. She's pulling at her ears.

I'm gonna get a gun and kill the SOB. We tried Tylenol.
My teeth, oh God. Bless you darlin'. *Squeeze my fingers,*
release. There are no more pillows. Everything off but panties
and socks. Does it hurt if I push here? Pee in this cup.

Don't shove that in my nose. I crawled to the phone. Call my
doctor, now. I'm cold. I can't stop shaking. Why do I need
a monitor? *Try this IV. I've stuck him twice. Call Rape Crisis.*
Did they tell you she's retarded? Any numbness? Sharp or dull?

The bead's in his left nostril. Gases, room 6. This will be tight. Does anything make the pain go away? Does anything make the pain better? Does anything make the pain go away? Squeeze my fingers, release, release.

Kindness

I'm not supposed to tell you this, but after report, there were nights, afternoons, days we'd lean over, whisper to each other (old church ladies gossiping), *If there's a rape tonight, I don't think I can do it.* And with our eyes, a pact was sealed. Bad stuff's cyclic, motorcycle wrecks on first warm days, GI bleeds at Christmas, autumn's flu. Our charge nurse could not suction trachs. She'd vomit. Right now. Right there. We knew, got her out of any mucus-gagging room. Because some of us birthed a stillborn, we'd say *If there's a SIDs baby, let Gina take the chest pains.* Or if people who are mislabeled as parents hurt a baby, (this could really get me in trouble) there are tubes and gizmos we'd like to demonstrate on them: Ewalds, defibrillators. But, our hands are busy, they are tied and after calling Children Services, we'd hear the CT was positive for a bleed (shaken baby syndrome/a kitchen counter fall?), by then a *I Just Graduated With My Masters* counselor paces near the station, stacks of forms you can barely see her lost-look eyes; experience is an empty backpack waiting in her car. She doesn't know how little people serve time, how the wrong people get a life sentence. These counselors fly solo, and human beings have limits. When someone says *sky,* your bullshit meter should have a seizure. Nurses memorize counselors' names, clear a patch of counter near a phone, show them where the bathrooms are so they can vomit in private.

The Language of Patients

Wrapped inside a sail of damp sheets
the baker's wife speaks only Italian now
—her stroke has rowed her home—
it's a salty lullaby, a toddler's fevered crib song.

Good morning Maria, I say,
I'm Susan, your nurse.
In her palms, I fix my fingers
squeeze with all your might, I tell her.

The temple of the self is silk.
I want my speech to be
her blanket's soft pink neck
as I check pupils with penlight.

Like milk from a pail, blood spilt
in the loft, stealing sweet taste
of grapes, warm smell of bread.
I wonder about words like *hurt* and *paralysis*

her right side's asleep, and now, does what's left
search for the other like a lost glove?
All morning long *Maria Lucia Theresa Garcia*
bikes the stone streets of her village,

her good hand waves to Father Giorgio.
When she tries to pick her gown's blue flowers,
it makes the sound of a mother's apron
against the screen door, one breath before

she calls us to supper.

Rain

Summer nights after our shift
Marilyn, Theresa and I sit
the bench outside the ER.

We sip cold coffee, smoke,
watch the big dipper
refuse to burn out.

Stubborn as Sam Morgan's
stiff lungs coughing years
of mill dust. They will not die,

but cannot live. Can this
be the same sky that bowed
to Cleopatra? tormented Van Gogh?

We are nurses, not Shaman,
we whisper what we know.
Our daughters swim faster

than this moon, our sons' faces
are passengers in train windows,
every half second, science invents

gizmos for us to memorize,
red alarms, green beeps, chants
to raise the dying. We are plain

gray doves that will fly
from this bench the way tide
leaves the shore. Others will come,

sponges to bathe the lonely,
webs to bandage the angry.
One day, we will leave

this world, overnight
we'll become the rain.

When My Brother-in-law Has Lung Cancer

The phone rings, my sister in California saying her husband's
been asking for ice cream, but she's changed both their diets
salads, fruits, everything healthy, and now, he's got diabetes
(not the needle, but it's looming), and she wants to do
the *right* thing. They told her the tumor's the size of an orange.
His chemo's been started. I talk to Kenny briefly, he's winded,
too tired for long distance anything. I ask my sister for her
work phone number, and she's so off her game, my request
seems benign. The next day, I drink my tea and pray.
I call her desk, listen, I say, I'm in Ohio, you're there, but I
think this: take a family leave, get a tub of ice cream, give him
two spoons, next week he may not be able to say what he wants,
from what you've told me (I take a big breath, blow it all out)
he may only have eight weeks. She starts to cry. Me too.
I want our Mom, for her, for me. California
is the other side of the world, and it's nobody's fault.
It's oat cell carcinoma, and he doesn't smoke anymore, just
retired, a good guy who volunteers at the conservancy.
Their plans to travel and camp get loaded in God's pickup,
but she gets her leave, and finally, so does he.

Long Distance

The woman on the phone talks with her friend in Myrtle Beach.
Next week: vacation, ten days, two couples, a visit with Ruth and Joe.
It's Thursday; it's garbage night, just now, dusk. The dog's asleep,
dreaming on a rug, so when her husband opens the kitchen door, gray
as a weathered fence saying, *I don't know what's wrong, but I didn't
think I'd make it back to the house*, she knows. She knows it's not
that far to their driveway's mouth and the can he carried was half
full. She knows right now their life's on fire, not a big flame, something
electrical in the cellar, something smoldering, doing its deed in darkness.
She reads his face like a newspaper, and haunting faces rise before her,
years of nursing men/women, they walk toward her like field hands
after the hottest August days. They're out of breath from pushing wooden
carts piled high with their good hearts, red as apples, everywhere in her
kitchen, the sweet smell of rot. How fast can she give an aspirin, a Nitro,
grab her keys and load him in the car? All the way to the ER they barely
speak, but what's twenty minutes in a lifetime? The Grand Canyon's down
the road. At the ER, she lifts the red phone, *My husband's a cardiac patient.*
She does not know the voice spilling out like pills on the counter. They
need a plan, a way to escape, but he's all wired up and looks *sick* in that
flowered gown. How many tests will he pass/fail? *In my top drawer*, he
says, *there's a pair of earrings for Summar* (our daughter) *for Christmas.* She
studies the floor and tells him she has to go pee. A lie. How many women
cry in bathroom stalls? She washes her face, opens a stick of gum. Day
three, the cardiac cath shows two blockages in the Widow Maker. He gets
two stents. She thought it was her day off. She thought it was Thursday.
She believed it was Ruth on the phone, but it was God, and when He asked
for her husband, she lied, she told God, *Sorry, he's not home.*

What Grief Is

For Sara & Florence

My sister's phone voice is a fist knocking on God's door,
                she has brought Him her best apple pie.

We've got an awful sick little girl here tonight she says.
(Her daughter, thirty-four, mother of three, melanoma).

Tell me what's going on, I sigh (sometimes love's
the black phone we must answer, my blood is theirs).

She has a terrible headache, a headache that won't go away.
Sara, get Flossie in the car now, I say, you and Randy

take her to the emergency room now, she needs a CT scan.
All right. I'll call you later. She hangs up and I wait. I want

to burn my scrubs, unlearn my twenty-five years of bedside nursing,
trade it back to be a lady bank teller, a schoolteacher with a room

full of eager faces, but midstream, there's no switching your wagon.
At the cutting-edge med center (a study Flossie was part of), the young

doctor says, *In her brain, more tumors than we can count.*
For a week, Flossie slept, and then the angels came, but not before

her nine-year old asked me *Aunt Jeanne, is Mommy going to die?*
My life's hardest question was a line drive, and I'd left my glove at home.

My sister, brother-in-law, Flossie's brother, sister, her precious girls,
her dear Randy, all of us? We poured Cheerios, packed lunches, got

little girls through Christmas, tried to fill in cold blanks of a million
spaces. Flossie's girls said their prayers, pasted *Have you seen my Mom?*

snapshots to their hearts' small walls. The pearl necklace of childhood
was broken, its jewelry box put away, something else took its place,

forever, in our chests, and the ball comes when we're not ready,
                it hits and hits and hits.

What Nurses Know

There is nothing stronger
than a child
and a needle in the same room.

I Will Breathe and Breathe

While the doctor says *bone tumor*
I will watch his nurse take you away for more x-rays.
You are five years old, my daughter. Your father's golfing.
I will blink and remember a one-legged woman skiing on TV.
I will change the words *chance of malignancy* to *mild blue skies*.
The hump on your scapula is cauliflower.
The lump on your left leg, a frond.
You are a bowl of petals, and this, an awful wind.
I will burn the doctor's tumor book; we'll run
from this office not knowing our destination.
I will tell your father a story about a wolf and a lamb,
a gate we did not close.
In the waiting room, children bald from chemo.
Your father's face hidden behind a magazine.
Your dolly's yarn hair, body of cloth, any flame
can take us. I will promise the tumor doctor
to harvest his thistle fields barehanded.
I will quit swearing. I will donate a kidney.
I will baby-sit the neighbor's retarded sons
while they visit Europe, Australia, Mars.
The doctor lifts you to his exam table, touches skin
where bone cells rage, drunken thugs in a cave.
When he says your name, it feels like calico,
soft and ready to be cut.

Birch Canoe

for Captain Dan Suttles

After supper, my daughter asked me,
Any bad stuff today?

I would like to tell her *no*,
but she's seen the six o'clock news,
yellow tape surrounding the trailer's shell,
the story of sisters playing with matches
our fire captain, tired, begging parents
to put lighters up, install smoke alarms.

She knows the child named Sara
came to my hospital.
I am touched by her concern,
Will they make it, Mom?

I try to tell her about the fireman,
young and sweaty and mustached,
his scorched suit
kneeling beside our gurney,
holding swollen sooty fingers
of a toddler he did not know,
praying for this flower he'd gone
into the flames to gather.

I try to tell her
about men who are gentle and strong,
men who rise without hesitation,
become larger than themselves
and do not paint their faces
with arrows and do not thump
their chests blue.

I do not know
how they tell themselves not to be afraid,
how they let the black smoke
swallow them over and over.
I just know tonight this fireman

was a birch canoe; he swam into the fire
and pulled Sara back into this world,
that is never easy.

Comfort

Nurses don't care when the coffee was fresh,
if it's one step above motor oil, hand it over
and no one will be hurt. Sorry to bring up our needs
first. Must be this shift I signed on for as a new graduate
thinking (of course) what would be best for my son/husband.
Me? Driving home, I doze off, windows down, white snow
hitting my face, 2 fresh sticks of Juicy Fruit spill sugar grit
roof to floor; still I nod and yawn. No warm spot waits,
but I enter my bedcovers like a lover. You see sleep deprivation's
the head nurse of every unit and her smoky kisses prick patients,
families and staff, but let's not speak of misery when white roses
sing at the station (Dawn let her husband move back home),
and those twin babies with gastro finally had a soft formed BM.
Yes, nurses rejoice over mushy moves because poop is good.
Sometimes, it means things are moving in the right direction.
Tonight we've forty-two tykes on Peds (twenty with IV's),
and four-year-old Amy calls from her 3 AM crib,
Doctor, doctor, help me. I have to pee.
Three admissions waiting in ER (pneumonia, croup, a hot appendix,
our charge nurse getting over a hyster, so I've got the desk, and respond
without an ounce of shame): Amy, *I'm coming.*
This is your nurse, Joanne. I am not the doctor. The doctor is home.
He is home in bed.

For the Nurse in Jackson Hole, WY, Who Cared for My Husband

for Mary Jo, ICU nurse

There you were, *Mary,*
    blinds behind you
        slats of darkness
            slicing light,

My husband's good heart
    rocking up and down
        on the screen's gray porch.
        He has asked the neighbors
            to sit a spell.

Each breath counts
    for something
        peaks and valleys,
            oxygen, a finger's pink
            measured like lemonade
            sold by small girls
                under a maple tree.

In the fog of morning
    we have traveled
        to this high place,
            you from a Minnesota farm,
                me from the projects of Ohio.

A blanket shawl drapes your shoulders
    as you hang each bag of blood,
        tiptoe in and out of his room.
            Mary, Mary, your young face bright
            with worry, your arms row
                three of us through such a hard night.

This cot you gave me
    becomes a sidewalk over a grate.
        I am a bag lady
            without boots or shoes
                a woman who sleeps in clothes.

III

Now is the time to be mute.
I will sit beside you without speaking.

I will cushion your bones in silence.
I will put my ear to your ear

and wait to hear a wave's scant echo
rippling from the distant rim.

-Alice Cone
"A Time To Be Mute"

Blue Kimono

Yellow metal carts sit in hospital
hallways and guard the doors.
Like clay lions they stay put
under a red sign that says
Stop, please see the nurse

before entering. For many reasons
a patient's door may be closed,
and on the other side, nurses
in gowns, masks and gloves
stay busy tending an Asian

grandmother. They change dressings
and hang fresh IV's. From the TV,
a spring shower of violin music.
The belly's incision yawns like
its zipper's been pulled down

exposing gray flesh, a foul odor
rises, but the grandmother smells
only herbal tea. Her mother pours
and pours it into glazed rosette cups.
Using a pink swab, one nurse cleans

night's prayer from the quiet tongue.
Worried, the respirator sighs. The doll's
eyes open, but fail to focus on the nurses'
ballet. Though the music's beautiful
and the dancers skilled, small hands lie
swollen, unable to clap. The voice

is a wren worn out from flying inside
a well. For a while the body's light
maintains its brilliance, but when
its song begins to fade, black notes
struggle to swim upstream. The nurses?
They comb and braid a girl's silk hair;

carefully, they tie her blue kimono.

Surgical Floor:
Student Nurse, Working for Pay, 1977

Report's folded like a note, but much heavier
in your left pocket. Eighteen patients to walk;
busy treatments, dressing changes, drains to empty,
call lights and pain. At the hall's end, good news,
a grandfather's going home, you push the wheelchair;
he's shaking hands with the guy in the next bed,
saying something about luck. When you come back
to strip his bed, the old man's roommate (thirty-one,
lung cancer, twin boys) needs to talk. His flood of bad
news today, no surgery will help; it's spread so far already
and *I wanted to see my boys play football. I wanted to see
my twins grow up.* He's just the age of your cousin
who likes to hunt and fish. Behind thick glasses, hazel eyes
float a gray pond. Down deep, someone's hook he's trying
to cough up. You are twenty-six, stuffing dirty sheets into a
blue linen bag, a sack big enough for Santa's toys. Maybe this
guy will not see Christmas. What rises in your throat is Dylan
Thomas' *Do not go gentle into that good night.*
He wants to coach his sons, make love to his young life.
(Who can blame him?) You lotion both hands, rub his back,
recite Thomas, because that's the lily in your other pocket,
and maybe it is grace.

Everyone in the Room Is Needed:
Clinical Rotation, Labor & Delivery, 1979

I didn't know how to act around doctors, afraid my words/
questions might sound dumb; I saved them for nursing
professors or looked them up later by myself. I was so
happy just to be learning so much so fast, getting a chance
for a seat at that table, breathing the same air as seasoned
obstetrical nurses, I thought washing our hands in the
same sinks, their knowledge might float up, touch my
forearms, and my veins would take it in like a sponge.
That morning, seeing my first birth, a caesarian section,
my heart was a bluebird bursting inside my chest, flying
against my rib cage with wonder. A beautiful almond-
skinned princess, her head a crown of soft black curls
appeared like the sweetest fruit from her mother's belly.
I cried standing on the periphery of the deck craning
my neck to see what the real nurses did. For most of the
case, I stood back, watching the movement of a strange
hand-and-eye ballet. The doctors and nurses passed silence
like instruments with their eyes, and until the needle count,
it was flawless. One needle missing, the doctors could not
close. Topside, on her trays, one nurse shook her blood-
stained gauze, counted sponges. The world stops without
that curved needle. Our hearts beat and the second hand
sweeps over its numbers, blood pulses through our veins,
the princess gets moved to the nursery, but the surgery can
not proceed. On my hands and knees, my eyes move like
a flashlight's beam for anything shiny, and after several
minutes, I found their needle like a button popped off in
the snow. One doctor said something like, *Well it wasn't*
a total waste of time having a student in the room. Without
contaminating the field, I struggled to get up and hand off
the needle. I can see the baby's small fists opening like
rosettes and hear her voice filling our room with joy.
What the doctor said or thought can't touch the bluebird
flying inside me now. I was trying to rise up
out of a life of being forever on the floor.

ICU Nurse Preceptor, 1981

This is the fairytale's middle part,
a bloodroot clearing surrounded
by a grove of trees
a place where someone's dragged the wounded.

Take a breath, take a minute, go slow, she tells me.

One of the good fairies,
she knows years of spells
under this bright noise
her brown eyes shine.

Something beeps, look at your patient, check equipment,
follow cords to the outlet.

Listen, the body's working class,
blue collar, no union. Hearts
cannot negotiate bereavement,
lungs don't get sick time or vacations.

This is the cottage
where the witch lives, these sons
and daughters followed her crumbs.
Like dough rising, some of the bodies swell.

Whatever swords they carried
were surrendered at the jamb,
even royalty, even the dark-skinned man
wearing his gauze turban,

two puffed eyelids painted purple,
his sorrel horse has left him.
I'm wearing my uniform and shined shoes.
She hands me a paper mask.

You might need this, she says walking me
to the door. *This is the burn pit,* she points,
throw everything in it before you go home.
If they ask, tell your family 'my day was fine.'

I'm learning to lie.
I'm memorizing my first spell.

The Delicate Cycle:
Being a Critical Care Nurse

There's no *excuse me* here, we are not women/men bumping into each other in the produce aisle, my winter coat doesn't brush your sleeve as we enter/leave the bank. After this week, we will not be neighbors. I won't get to tell you how your husband looked standing there by the wall facing your machines like a firing squad. No blindfold, both his hands bound with love. Above your gown's blue flowers, I'm a worker bee; our queen's got the desk. Me? I hover, weave and fly. I listen, suction, bag, calibrate, measure, lift and turn write down every living secret. Those busy wings? My chapped hands. They hang blood, heparin saline and Dopamine from metal poles like diapers on a renter's porch. Sorry, no geraniums, no window boxes, just a neon moon, crated, boxed and glued to our ceiling. Caught in trauma's hammock, the gods let you sleep and dream. You're just the age of my Mama when she died, but I won't tell you that. Do you mind the wind of so many bodies passing night and day? As our ballet of warm cloths soap and rinse, I'm the beggar behind pain's fence, *Marge, please stick out your tongue.* Familiarity amid this noisy rain. Beeps, sighs, scratchy sheets, but I have this yellow lotion for your back. Sorry about your wedding band. The body swells. I had to. Yes, that's me saying, *Now boarding at Gate Six* (nurses also need to smile), and four of us will lift you to a recliner. The yank on your catheter? Not me. We can't be on both sides of the bed. The pillowcase folded like a scarf to hide the egg-shaped drain? Me. (Your kids don't need to see it). When I'm at break, the neurosurgeon gets his shorts all bunched up, and my charge nurse takes the heat for your babushka. Surgeons. You wonder if they had a Mom. Get the bleach. We're not to bad mouth colleagues, because on this block, we all run out of sugar, need coffee passed over the fence. Ask our cleaning lady; Ruby has her Ph.D. in muck and suds. Across the bays we call to each other, women/men in scrubs. Hard to believe all the wash we've taken in, so many years of lights and darks.

In the Dirty Utility Room, ICU 1982

for Myrtle

This room's small, cluttered, the white sink's deep
lots of water, a nozzle to rinse, a handle to flush.
Today's odor's melano, bloody feces, I'm emptying

a bedpan for the fifth time when Myrtle appears
dragging her linen sack, her black faces shines
circled by those gray curls, and her gold cross

sleeps above her breasts. And nobody says, *Lordy,
Lord* but Myrtle after cardiac arrests and the hoop-la
of reinserting chest tubes.

Miss Jeanne, she says, *I'm glad you're feeling better.
I'm glad you're on the other side.* How'd she know?
You never told her, the infertility clinic, 150 miles

three times a week, all these months, all the money.
The baby you both wanted, but will never have.
She hugs you. *I watch my nurses;*

I know when my girls are hurtin'.
And for one moment, her arms around you are a quilt,
she's your Mom, her soft body's a pillow, in her lap

you sleep, this train pulls away from sadness.
Two women, and every hard mile
you've both traveled to get here, to lay your face

on Myrtle's sweet chest, to empty your heart's gravel.
What would you give to stand with her,
now by her stool, where after a Nitro,

she sometimes sat alone till the pain eased?
*Miss Myrtle, I'm glad you're feeling better.
I'm glad you're on the other side.*

Assessment

If you see wrist scars
kneel down,
check both ankles
offer to wash her feet.

Violets

In the hospital's emergency room
there's a girl with enormous
eyes and shoe string hair
who puts razor blades on her tongue,
in her vagina, across her wrists
month after month.

She lives in a country
where there are no prophets.
our longest bridge of candles
will not lift her to the ridge
over this black river.

Any meadow needs flowers in it
or a small girl dragging a red sled
while her dog jumps beside her.
A child wants cocoa waiting,
dry socks folded on the bed.

Consider this girl,
saving her razors like ticket stubs.
What makes her believe
the razor's kiss can heal a life
battered as a sparrow?

Nights they bring her to us,
dull as a gray rag, we wash her
the way you'd wash a mauled terrier.
And when we close her skin
with suture, scars blossom pink scrolls

—rows of azaleas—like nothing
you can smell or taste, like little girls
in their eyelet sundresses
running toward you
their fists full of violets
crying, *Here, here, love me.*

HS Care

Loneliness has no cure.
Nurses warm the lotion,
tenderly rub its bony spine
and red coccyx.

Afternoon Shift, 1979

Warm and black, the night's fuzzy arms
wrap around hospital windows, in a breezeless town
lights twinkle. A nurse, I think of orderly women
busy at home, nursing infants, checking fractions,
making love to their blue collar husbands.

Pink-gray smoke settles in our sky, heavy breath
from the mill's nostrils, an aging workhorse,
his coarse hair full of burrs. I shake plastic pitchers,
wonder how much life is spent in eight hours?

Stuck to an old guy's buttocks, we find a silver spoon.
I thought I felt something down there, he says.
We laugh and shake our heads. Lucky for him,
for us, his skin's not torn. My lotioned hands rub
and rub. Mary lifts his glasses, gentle, gentle, she

says his name. Mr. Lincoln smiles, pulls out
his dentures. A round lid fastens. His tall body's
the color of fallen chestnuts, long arms like my papaw.
What does our laughter mean? This slice of quiet,
the teaspoon we've found and freed?

The urine's warmth gathered like gold?
Given time, we'll make our mark.

Was that the lesson for today?

Dear God,

Just wondering if You heard Janet last night when she was getting her jacket, cramming her stethoscope in the locker, ready to collapse? Did You hear her response when I said, "You look so tired?" *Because I am. Because I've worked two doubles and I'm doubling back for day turn tomorrow.* You must have seen my hand go to her shoulder when I asked, "Why, why are you doing all these shifts?" *So many are off sick and vacations. There's nobody else.* Lord, look at her back, how it aches under the weight, her ribs starting to show. You have the ledger: a house burned, a divorce, both breasts are taken, her husband lost his job and can't find work. No wonder she's the same color as the gray locker. She's fifty-seven, but study her forehead leaned against the metal locker like it's a gun, a gun she almost wants, but cannot hold, sleepy drunken words spill from her lips. She's not really fit to drive home. It's true she's a fighter, that farm accident, thrown from her horse cost her a hip, but how many lathered runs can a mare stand spring upon spring? Her paycheck's the family well. Insurance keeps her stabled in this stall. Our cavalry, the new nurses, can't ride fast enough to save us all. And those fresh fillies and stallions leave in herds. Inside the barn's blaze, they refuse to be silent, won't be trampled under hooves of paperwork. Won't lift a shovel for someone else's manure. They aren't signing on for thirty, forty years of a loveless marriage, won't mortgage their lives to save others. So when Janet says *there's nobody else* she's speaking gospel. We both know working like Clydesdales won't get us anywhere but dead. I should have grabbed Janet's keys, but You know, I am a coward, still working part time. Lord forgive me, being lame, it's the best I can do.

Silence Gives Consent

Bargaining with hospital management
to stop mandatory overtime, get a decent raise,
make sure patients really do come first has hit a wall,
so when the strike notice has been sent, when you clock out
knowing supervisors and head nurses will be spread mighty thin
for patients who could not be discharged, you see ants
in a new way, understand how they can move a slice of bread.

One November, two weeks over the burn barrels, sharing the night fire
with brothers and sisters, you grew taller, sat a little straighter
in your kitchen chair, because (after all these years) nursing unions
had a turn with the ball, after 8 or 10 or 12 hour shifts, sometimes
you hardly know your name let alone how to mix and titrate five drips
for one patient. You aren't sure if your feet will carry you to your car
in the lot (Which gray four-door is it?).

Thank goodness your car knows the way home, and tonight,
on the neuro-spine unit, when it was just you and Beth, 2 RNs
for 18 patients (my hand to God), and that direct admit post-op
laminectomy woman screaming in agony, her back swollen
clear to her bra line, writhing like a worm on pain's hook,
when you'd stuck her twice for an IV (both veins blew),
when her aunt, a retired nurse, whispered

Let me, I'll never tell. You wanted to kiss her, and your heart
did a happy dance when her family said *we're staying all night.*
God is good, you say to yourself walking
to the station, in room 555, tonight, my patient has a chance.

Nurses Stand Up for Healthcare Reform

Mr. President, Speaker of the House, Senators, Congressmen,
I ask the chair to recognize the delegates standing in scrubs.
No sir, we did not fly on private jets. We car-pooled.
Yokes? Yes sir, the draped stethoscopes are symbolic.
Yes sir, we are tired. Coffee would be nice.
No sir, donuts are not necessary, but the bathrooms?
Thank you. Thank you very much.
The speaker calls on Urgent Care.
Thank you Mr. President, Mr. Speaker, Senators, Congress.
I make a motion that when a guy lacerates two fingers, his thumb
in a machine and he's working for less than minimum wage,
driving a 1987 Lick-and-a-Promise, barely enough money
for gas, wearing work boots that wouldn't pass for flip-flops,
apologizing for bleeding on the sheets, and I know he has
to spend the five dollars he's got (counting change) for milk
and bread, I make a motion there's a pharmacy he can go to
get his antibiotic and five pain pills with a voucher.
I move that if this motion isn't drafted and passed,
all the grunts who end up having hand surgery (which costs
$50-80,000) and lose the use of their dominant hands
be made wards of the state and get to live (wife, kids, dogs and all)
in the governor's mansion for free. Thank you.

IV

On the outside, and on the inside too, my house is falling down.
This is the blue house that came after the white house
with yellow shutters, the one we expect to live in
for the rest of our lives.

-Hope Gilliam
"How the End Came"

Mercy

This grandmother I'm holding the phone for lives on
a pension of chalk and ashes; tonight walking to the grocery,
a van hit her, kept going. A man (she said it was a white man)
left her, a snapped branch out in the cold, honking rain. I mean
lying near a storm sewer with two broken legs isn't like sitting
at a counter, reading the blackboard's menu deciding what we want,
what we'll settle for if they're out of tomato bisque. Even at dusk,
there's no mistaking a woman's shape for crumbs, our ice bags negate
piles of warm blankets. Who knew her husband was just discharged?
Heart attack, legally blind. They are both crying. *I love you. I'm so sorry,*
please take your pills, on the counter by the toaster, yes, I will try
to call Ted, I don't know. I know, don't, please, don't cry.
Here, talk to the nurse, she knows.
But, I don't. I don't know when her surgery will be or how her legs
will heal. I don't know if she'll get pneumonia or blood clots. There's a
risk. That's what I know. I know she wears the quiet face of kindness,
and this room's bloated with noise. I know this phone is black, we're
at the station, my feet ache and she needs the pain shot she won't take.
I want to believe she will get well enough to go home, fill his pill pods,
wash his back. Like me, they have a life, a house where the roof slopes,
so the rain and snow won't come in, maybe peonies border her porch.
In my pocket, there's a scratch off ticket for long shots. I saw a penny
in her purse. That's what I know.

Body Mechanics

Those football-player guys dressed in scrubs
at big city clinics, between lifts,
what do they do? We have seen their biceps
and thighs pressed against navy blue cotton.

Aaah. Charleton Heston's bare arms
in the Ten Commandments. And we know
we should not covet, but untangling women's legs,
men's shoulders (a full arrest or gunshot wound),

straddling crumpled bodies on the car's floor,
(backseat of a two-door), opening an airway,
(blanched tongue clenched in teeth),
one of us starting compressions,

dragging folks to gurneys like shot deer,
(our own guts unfastening in the process),
small community hospitals, year after year.
Laminectomies, hysterectomies, bladder suspensions,

total knees. Miles nurses travel before we rest.
Oh lift Brothers, where art thou?
From a far place, we ached for your arms,
dreamed of you as stars.

We will let you meet our surgeons;
we will let you count our scars.

When a Friend Asks Me What It's Like to See Someone Die

for Brian

Maybe because I'm a nurse
and his mother weakens as her cancer spreads,
he wants to know the path of beautiful stars.

He needs to understand trajectory, but the loft
I paint stretches between the nave and choir,
a brown altar boy with dreds

barely fourteen, shot with a handgun near his thigh.
In the chapel of crash carts, sirens and bells,
we lift, roll, scrape red and sew

work on him like a canvas, palm his chest like clay, like dough.
This Bob-Marley boy fallen asleep in his Father's chair.
This Nigerian prince quiet from poison's dart.

This child who chases a balloon through night's park
                             his eyes hungry for wonder.

Forgiveness

I.
Dr. Brown wears his black wing tips, navy blue suit, *After Life*
cologne and his wavy white hair. He's tall as a rocket, and I want
to ask him where he splashed down after his cancer, but I don't.
We're in my cellar, wooden beams, cobwebs, painted block walls.
I continue to pull warm clothes from the dryer, a big load of darks.
Surgeons, I shake my head, when you need one they're never near.
But here we both are, last load of the day and Dr. Brown just appears
between pillow cases and my full-figured bras (the lace ones) hanging
from a metal line. He watches me unscrew the bulb over the washer.
My flip-flops whisper against the cement, and like a dance partner,
he follows my lead. I almost apologize for the workbench mess,
the sprung mousetrap.

II.
Upstairs, he seems tired; I nod him toward my husband's recliner. I'm
a little surprised when he sits. I dump the basket on the couch. *You're
all dressed up,* I say and wonder if those are his burying clothes. "Yes,"
he tells me, "it's my favorite suit." The snap on my daughter's jeans
briefly burns my thumb. Our dog, always glad for company, jumps
up, licks Dr. Brown's long fingers, sniffs his crotch. *Sorry,* I cringe
(half-smiling). "The way you toss and fold those towels," he praises.
For a moment, I stop my work. *Why are you here?* I ask. *No golf?*
"Not today," he sighs. The dog takes off with a dryer sheet, and I
lunge to snatch it back. Our living room's not the place for Dr. Brown,
my husband's big wrench mounted on oak (a retirement gift from his
coworkers), our kids' graduation photos, my grandmother's ivory
Bible.

III.
"That Tuesday in the OR," he begins. *When I was a student?* I cut in.
"Yes." *And they switched the order of your cases?* (I want to be sure).
"Yes." *And you'd just told your golf-partner friends they'd be able to
see their son in recovery, a hernia repair's almost like peeling an apple?*
"Yes." *And then you walked in on that fifty-six year old woman already
under for her gall bladder, a diabetic?* "Yes." *And you went 'Jesus Christ,
somebody get their ass upstairs and talk to those parents. Who the hell
brought her down' crazy?* "Yes." *After you left, for those five minutes,*

they were nearly peeing their pants, thought they'd have to reverse the
woman, do the hernia kid first. "No." *Yes. They were really scared. Me*
too. I was the only student in the room. "I remember." *You do?* "Yes,"
he points to my legs, "your white hose." *Why did the real nurses put me*
in your armpit for first assist? He shrugs. *Well, I didn't know a Deaver*
retractor from a Phillip's screwdriver. For almost three hours your
tongue was my scalpel. You screamed your way through layers of fat and
fascia, finally pulling what was rotten out.

IV.
(I put my hand on my hip and talk loud for this part): *You think*
I didn't know how fast you had to change your game plan?
That you looked the fool for one moment?
He rubs his eyes, studies his hands, my bifocals.
"I'm sorry," he says, "I'm really sorry." All the while he pets
and pets Belle.
Coffee? I offer.
"Sure," he says as he struggles to stand, "and show me where
the towels go."

Where They Live Now

When I knock, Patsy comes to the door, her shock of curly red hair tied back. *Hey you, give me a hug*, she says. "The others?" *Those bums sleep late.* "For all of you," I say, handing her yellow daisies. Our coffee's black, strong. "Who plays?" I nod toward the keyboard, drums, two guitars. *All of us*, she says. "Really? I never knew." *Before, we didn't, but here, it's different, and the Stones have fifteen years on us, so why not?* "Indeed," I say. Some laundry drapes the porch rails, white scrub dresses, lab coats, shirts. "The stories about robes, wings?" *Not true*, she says as she lights up a smoke. "You were a great head nurse." *I was all right.* "They've done away with Peds, but we've got a union now." *I know.* She takes a long drag, rubs her shoulder. "Does it still hurt, where the melanoma started?" *No, not really.* I hear the others starting downstairs: Roseann, Marsha, Trudy. In a circle, we laugh and cry. There's much to say and I've only the morning. They wear panties under the band's black T-shirts **Five Hearts**. "Why an extra heart?" I ask. *Because the one they gave me didn't work*, Trudy yells over the blender. "Your cottage reminds me a bit of Ireland so lovely here by the sea." Marsha sighs, *At first, I wasn't sure about being by the water, you know, drowning sucks.* Roseann goes to her, tries to change the subject. *We built this place ourselves.* "Therapy," Patsy says. *Pink-ribbon anger management*, Roseann smiles. The hotcakes are sloppy with butter and syrup. "I was a little surprised by the lane's distance," I say, "though it's a peaceful drive, and peaches ready to pick in May." *Seasons are endless here*, Trudy says, *but some neighbors complain.* "About peaches?" *No, we practice late*, she goes on, *mostly it's the docs: no lit tennis courts, no ear plugs here. All night long they still have to listen to us.*

Last Trees

When fog lifts in the farmer's field,
have you seen those last trees
standing like a brick chimney
after a house fire?

The gnarled oaks and maples
whose limbs beg for sky?
They're the bald men in sweaters
sons/daughters wheel to ER
saying, *He seems fevered, can't pee*

maybe three days. Nurses wrap
both arms around their trunks,
pivot dingy undershirts and seasoned
smell of flesh to gurneys.
We unzip trousers, lift thin arms

through flannel sleeves. (How is it
they are *cold* in July/August?)
We thread and tie the gowns,
place blue flowers on writhing
bodies of brown leaves.

Their swollen bellies hold melon
prostates and maybe cancer's seed.
For living a long life, men receive
a key to the basement apartment,
torn curtains and bad plumbing.

When we swab their penises
with betadine, pass special
catheters dipped in gel, when
the body's honey starts to flow
and their breathing begins to slow

as both fists relax, birds fly faraway.
And the men? These beautiful old trees?
Their eyes say,
May the angels lead you into paradise.

Colonoscopy:
Encouraging Patients to Vent

It's just air, we tell them, but many are bashful
as lilies especially middle-aged men, the ones
who still wear white briefs.

While I scoop their clothes, take their vital signs,
I'm Katie Couric asking *how was the prep? Able
to drink it all? Your last movement, what color was it?*

If you walk in shy, you'll leave proud because we're
not talking The Price is Right; this is Survivor. The island
fills and empties with new members of the pineapple brotherhood.

You can imagine the gut's surprise, mid December waking
a brown bear in his den. You weren't expecting a stick of dynamite
lit and thrown. And now, your body says *Come on down,*

you're bathroom king for a day. One man felt called
to witness (I swear), he said I read three Playboys, one Smokey
Mountain knife catalog and two Reader's Digests before the muskets

slowed, and I had time to think between magazines, time to make
a plan. *Go on*, I said. Well, after I scrubbed the john, I got myself
showered and shaved. When I thought it was safe, I dressed. I nod.

I went to the cellar, took down my gun, two shells and loaded both
barrels. In the kitchen, I grabbed the plastic jug by its neck, swung
it like a duck, stood it on a backyard stump, blasted it to Kingdom
Come.

That, he said, felt like justice.

Now You Know

You sit in a recliner at the infusion clinic, and your nurse, Howard, (did you really just say that?) washes his hands like a surgeon before he starts the IV. The medicine takes four hours to infuse, he says. (Your right eye, auto immune arthritis, loss of vision). Nervous, you keep talking, I feel fine, just can't read a thing on the eye chart with this eye, it's like someone wrote in magic marker and then it rained on the letters. Howard listens, rips tape, opens the needle package. He has to stick you twice (what? you always said, I have Ray Charles-Stevie Wonder veins). Smartass. Now, see where you're sitting? Who cares if it was just a line you made up for those wild-and-crazy shifts in ER? You have just been converted. You are a witness for the pain scale. The 22 gauge needle digging the back of your hand? It's a "5," after Howard tapes it, a "1," when it's gone, a zero. Howard's got Chron's, he says MRSA, how he got it after an IV stick and it went to his valves; he ended up with open-heart surgery! He's so young . . . (how many times I've said that). He's so kind . . .(you think only mean people get aces and eights)? It's not fair . . . (show me justice and I'll show you fists in the air, faces shouting, point to streets where there's blood). I am writing in my journal, trying to read an article about fiction's point of view, some hot shot New York writer, but what if they can't fix my eye? Blake. I'll be Blake. Calm down. Howard's telling you to be careful about the IV site, (this medicine weakens immune systems and six pages of other stuff). The place where his needle went in, germs could find it, and it could be bad, like Howard, a helicopter ride, landing in open-heart country, the wide open spaces, the range with its endless sky.

Tuesday Night Special

For a long time you sit The Charmed Diner's third red stool. Fran knows you take one sugar, double cream and your fingers like the cup's weight, its flawless fired surface, the warmth and sweetness of what's inside. Newspaper stories you read waiting for hash browns, eggs over easy and toast, gauntlets of faces, folks you've never met, here and there, fighting lost causes, waving adversity's flags, patterns of bullet spray, a house fire where a plane went down. Aren't they ulcers on the world's giant foot? Last week, your bowling partner's elderly brother got all jammed up when he ran naked down Oak Knoll claiming to be from Pluto. And Fran's crying, saying her son is into drugs. No wonder she forgot your ketchup. You were surprised just now by the obituaries, Carl's boy gone at thirty-five. Heart. And when Fran's finished, you give her your hanky, you don't jump on her raft, the brief suspension of her voice, because her wide, sad eyes remind you of your beagle, Slip, the gravel day he was hit, dying in the road, he'd lost a lot of blood and the old man wouldn't let your Mom take him to the vet for a good death. You're nearly sixty, and that open-faced sandwich is the Tuesday special you want someone to bring you (smothered with gravy) when it's your turn to give up this stool.

When Our Mothers Come for Us

I've seen it over and over, patients call 'Mom'
and lift both arms up in the air.
-Patty S., Hospice Nurse

In heaven, when Moms finish
painting their toenails hot pink
or watching General Hospital,
they sit on stars, legs dangling
barefeet slowly kicking back and forth.

Julia Child does all the cooking,
serves perfect meatloaf and baked
sweet potatoes on paper plates.
What a relief to not fret over
celery stalks getting slimy

in the crisper or dust bunnies
playing freeze tag under beds.
Aaah. No more smelly socks
or muddy jeans. No more squirting
blue stuff before scrubbing toilets.

But Moms miss us, and now they
pace in front of a huge elevator
like a bunch of high school girls
who've been shopping all day
for prom. Their young faces

aglow, voices praising their beautician.
She's given them all a *really good perm*.
In calico blouses or house dresses,
black stretch pants or not, they have
their instructions: fifteen minutes

to briefly go back. Pocketbooks over
their left forearms, they are coming for us—
slumped in a gray wheelchair, glazed
eyes staring straight ahead or thrashing
limbs sideways in a metal bed—

with rat-tail combs and brushes, their
wiping hankies pressed.
A thousand red-lipped kisses
for us to wear
and shirts that say,
You're gonna love it here.

Evening Prayer

for Dr. Zul Mangalji, physician and friend

Our bodies which art in decline
hallowed be thy buckled floors
dusty plaster of crumbling knees.
The projector room inside our temples
housing reels of dreams?
Blessed be its vista of colors, seascape
and pampas grass, monsters
slain by our Mothers' voices.

Blessed be this harvest
silver shocks found in our hair
sagging timbers of upper arms
the jaw's hammock.
Blessed be the parade
of brown spots giggling across
cheeks and nose. Plenty as nest eggs

we are yoked and speckled. Bless our breasts,
some cut away like roses, the rest
napping in our bras. Bless those nipples,
all electricity passed through them
free of charge. Bless also the bladder's
sonar, twilight's tow rope leading us
to the bathroom. Blessed be warm smell

of bean soup rising from the gut's kitchen,
blessed be the rumble of those pots and pans.
And the quiet barges inside our veins, tugs
returning dirty blood, valves opening
like locks? Hallowed be their red seas,
blessed be their captains. Give thanks
for once being able to run, making love

and call the ears' tiny bones home.
The foggy windows where memory stands,
small in her flannel gown, waving
to fast train of days, blowing kisses

to the moon? Blessed be this child's
blonde garland of curls
and welcome her one night
as the star she is into thy kingdom.

V

What notes can I leave on the kitchen table?
What blossoms?

-Katherine Orr
"After the Reunion, She Reads Her Diary"

For My Mother's Nurses

When I see wild white daisies stretching in grass, legions
of them waving near dusty country roads, I see mother's nurses.
I think, *Well, finally you all have slowed down, fixed a lemonade,*
found a porch swing and get to have a lazy day.
To work in a psyche hospital, lock-the-doors keys in your pocket
every day, well, it must feel a lot like carrying cement blocks. Not like
surgery where we pluck rotten apples from the barrel, close
the body's lid and go home. These bodies are cars that keep running
out of gas. They circle the block and head back to the station.
Our mother made things for us, once for me, a little crocheted cross,
a book mark for my Bible. Perhaps you remember her? In summer,
a blonde streak appeared like magic in her hair. It was a long time
ago. And I probably don't want to know the things you had to do
back then (in the 50's and 60's) to calm the seas of a manic cycle.
How many shots of whatever it was and how many people it took
to hold her down, making her mouth open like a pig for its apple
before the electro shock therapies. Whatever all that looked like,
I don't want to know. She had a red corduroy duster. Maybe you
helped her with its zipper 'cause many times her hands would shake.
Looking beyond your treatments, exhaustion and charting, I've
imagined you—aging faces of strangers, rows of beautiful nurses—
another scrapbook of a forgotten lot, flowers, white daisies coming
always to her bed, helping her down the halls, your voices a chorus
coaxing her to focus on the next step (whatever it was) to bring her
out of the foxhole and get her home (even a few days) to us.
Aunt Trudy sent her sky blue slippers. She cried for years over them.
A coffee stain. Maybe you saw it happen, one morning at breakfast
in the dining hall? Her hands did their dance and she'd wring them
when she paced the floor. She'd wring them like an old cloth full
of troubles. Over and over and over her sickness took her from us.
And then, for a while she was yours, because that's what nurses say,
She's my patient. In the land of the lost she appeared at your door
and you took her in like an orphaned child. You sewed patches
on her dress, combed her hair and made sure her letters got mailed.
You went home to your own hard chairs in this world. Writing
this note, please forgive its lateness (I was raised better). Saying
Thank you to nurses, who must surely be dead, folks will whisper.

They may say, *See, it runs in families; she's crazy as her mother.*
But, I'm not writing one phrase to them. I'm just saying
this is private—between nurses—to be here, you need a special key.

Blessing

I am writing this on a grain of rice.

Nurses are ants; this grass is wet, thick,
air smells like bleach over dirty socks.
Like crumbs, we carry our patients.
We are not priests. We are not rabbis.

This mission's no picnic,
pushing boulders alone,
wheeling hay bales to x-ray,
sorting and shoveling every kind of manure.

Those little mats the monks sit?
The oms they hum? Under our breath,
we curse and bless, then sip dark tea's
hard work. This ten-story hospital's

a gray lego in God's toy box.
We sift the language of pain, translate
dialects of suffering. Every patient carries
a *me first* card; they won't leave home without it.

And their phony-baloney meter's
always running, so beware.
Every shift we are held in the palm
of a hand we may never see.

Once, in ICU a woman woke from a coma,
laughed with her four kids, hugged them.
Her room was a village lit with love.
I saw that thirty-minute rainbow.

The next day, the woman was called home.
I dialed the black phone, told the husband,
bathed her, wrapped her in warm blankets.
When they came, I stood for her, for them.

Two of her girls grabbed on to me,
a rope to flailing arms, they wept, sobbed.
Our bodies melted together like candles,
their braids were petals of fresh shampoo.

It felt holy, like saying grace at my grandmother's table.

Breast Cancer Survivors:
Writing Workshop, One Thursday Night At Burger King

Because we'd been locked out of the art gallery
(a sculptor forgot to leave the key she'd slipped into her purse),
I said, maybe we should cancel class. (November, six women
huddled in one car, our breath steaming windows like we're
cooking soup). *No, no, no.* They chant it like a song rehearsed;
We've done our homework. "Okay," I say, "but where?"
Someone says, *Burger King.* We laugh. "Okay, meet you there."

At first the corner booth reminds me of crows, back and forth
catcalls, seven kids from *I don't give a shit* high school,
skull tattoos, spike dog collars, blue hair, every phrase
laced with *fuck* and *bitch.* I'm the workshop teacher.
I am well and start to wonder if what we're watching
might be the end product of a terrible experiment;
mold bubbling up from having it your way.

We get in line, buy our coffees. Two of the women smoke.
Class begins the old way, my tape recorder hums piano music,
ocean spray against a rocky shore, slow deep breaths.
Spiral notebooks open hymnals in our laps. And I like
how one woman gives her husband hell (roses sent
first time, after her breast was removed), how another
tells her kids not to be afraid in foster care, she hopes

they'll soon sleep under one roof. And God, well, She's
afternoon-turn shift leader in a hair net dressed like
somebody's Mom who'd really be pretty if she had teeth.
She's barking orders to the grunts in back and listening
very carefully to the real deal, the *No happy meals sold here* poets.

Their journal entries stab of biopsy needles, the physics
and bullshit of lugging a case of Ensure up two flights
of stairs, outside apartment, winter's ice, letters to lost breasts,
shock of being bald, endless puking after chemo.

You might not believe this,
but those kids in the corner booth?
They disappeared.

I don't know when,
but this really happened, just ask God.

The Elder's Circle:
Assisted Living Writing Workshop, 1999

If I look up, I can see her nervous smile,
Shady Rest's new activity director, summa cum laude
Mount Hickory University. Like a conductor's baton
her French nails wave the pen as she weaves in and out
of thirty-eight rooms asking *clients* what events they crave.

Her first job, she believes *patients come first*: active listening's
not rugby. She's a stewardess with a clipboard.
They are her passengers waiting to take off. They've raspy
answers to question number three: *What's your idea
for mornings at Shady Rest?* So far, six requests for poetry,

a poet, poems, someone to read Hiawatha, sonnets, the Raven.
Poetry? Are you kidding? She smells a rat. The balding orderly
on afternoons with his *Against the Wind* tattoo? Maybe.
Or the single Mother of twins who works laundry?
Rap, Dylan, she's heard both blaring from their junk cars.

Later, she scans the yellow pages, but nothing's listed
between moving Pods and A-Z Plumbing. What she must
have thought Googling poet: Frost, Dickinson, Yeats.
Dead, dead, dead. (tags you must tiptoe around on this job).
Tearful, she calls home, her Mom's romance novel club, they

meet at the bookstore next to Good Will. She dials the number.
Late afternoon, I get her message, can you come on Wednesdays?
We can't pay much (my usual fee). "Yes," I say, "I can do it." A poet,
a nurse, now, I'm part of the answer to question three. My small
tape recorder became a gray hive alive with stories: wedding

parties (Boston to San Francisco), a preemie son who fit
in a shoebox and lived! (before NICUs), boys/girls knitting
squares for WW I soldiers, a teacher who first earned $800/year.
For ten weeks each poet's song was a bird's shadow moving
across snow, a moonflower opening one last time, and me?

I was a cook boiling chicken for a rich man's table.
These cover girls dragged cobbled bodies to my soup kitchen.

Walkers, oxygen tanks and hose, shiny spokes of wheelchairs.
We shared salty broth of talk/listen, pointed to ache of joints,
named the quilt's pieces of pennies saved and spent.
They became speakers of the house. And even if I could coax
them back for one more summer; they'd not come.
Listen, please to Adela's:
Smelling the fire and feeling / the wind on your face /
the smoke, how it stays / in your hair and clothes / that's camping.

Why the Nurse Retired Early

So I might have time to visit the crater of thirty-four years,
bring this basket, gather petals and gravel, lint and leaf,
imagine mountains of sheets I've touched, washed,
hanging on a line, the morning's sunny, nobody's scared.

So I could go to my knees before my professors, women who wore
suits, men in ties who had the kindest eyes, a brilliance
that lit candles, invited me to their table, fielded endless questions,
steadied medicine vials for my trembling hands, the new passport

they handed me for my life, saying *How do you feel about that?*
(Like hey, are you talking to me?) The blue pie of critical thinking,
how they sliced it, how they shared.

So others could speak the truth about being in uniform
how we never got cookies from home
letters from girl scouts, how bullies pushed our cheeks
against the ground and we got up, to lift
the body bags, to load the choppers.

So I could wave a hanky of thanks to the doctors' wives
for picnic tables, the healing garden, an island of pink bushes,
butterflies—grace—caught between webs of oozing cases.
A place to stretch and listen and chew our life stories

like crackers and apples, tart juices drip from our chins.
So I might pass my map, tell new grads,
Your pin's a St. Christopher's medal,
take good notes; question what you do not understand.

Come to the table thinking where we might find water,
where we must drill new wells, how many acres should
be planted this year and the next. Part of nursing
is learning how to die and you may want to turn away,
but nothing must be forgotten.

Spared

The pretty nurse with all those initials behind her name
(almost an alphabet) is fretted up at the trauma conference,
her power point bullets too slow for her sermon. She says
her colleagues should not get giant fries, double whopper-
bacon cheeseburgers, mega Cokes, they must not reward
themselves after a multiple-vehicle call (a semi, three cars),
after picking up a girl's head from a ditch, a boy's arm near
a tree, a pregnant woman's body mashed through a steering
wheel, after holding sheets around all that so other freeway
drivers might be spared. After not crying or puking, not losing
it (almost never, maybe 20-30 years) she wants them to know
the better path is exercise. A big fireman sitting next to me sighs,
I pass him my cream stick. He smiles. Trembling with conviction,
she explains how we need a gym at every hospital (the fireman
chokes, I can't look at him), because as a flight nurse she goes
there: to bike, run, do a thousand crunches, walk her chained bear
on the treadmill so it will sleep. I think of my colleagues, the night
they had to identify two carloads of teens by their socks (with the
parents). I was not the nurse that night. I was not a mother screaming,
nodding *yes* to socks. I was not a father walking through fire holding
my son. The afternoon my friend's baby drowned? I was home weeding
zinnias, a meatloaf in the oven. People say they don't know how to
believe, but God is real. I have seen the work of His hands,
and I have felt His mercy.

On Blistered Walls

I have seen the body unhinged from itself like a barn's weathered door and in those moments following, I've heard its voice, knives sawing tin foil. And I have bathed the frozen tundra of catatonia, swabbed strep's raspy throat, patched together nasal syntax of the near deaf, marveled at the froggy vowels of a radical neck's laryngectomy. I have witnessed the teacher holding her chalk at the blackboard of old age, her eyes blank as the slate. Over the ribbed canyon of an open chest, I have leaned and watched the surgeon scoop hands full of clots to our ER floor. Yes, I can tell you blood turns to something between pudding and jello, smells metallic, and speaks the language of wet mops when it hits the tiles. I have followed orders and given commands. When the doctor tells me to insert large bore IVs in both feet, deep down, we already know our work's useless; behind these masks our faces belong to thieves. We are stealing moments, gloved hands held up in mid air, both barrels of this young face pressed to our chest. From ears, mouths, rectums, vaginas I have seen blood pour like a faucet, a faucet that will not be shut off. All of this I have beheld, and I have picked pockets, lifted wallets, turned myself into a little girl searching her Mother's Sunday purse for a stick of gum, for I needed the body's name, and many times its pockets were mute. Later, in years of quiet, I have come to the altar of my desk asking for words to paint what's sacred, those *up close* moments and *at the shift's end* and *now*, but for the most part, I'm still thumbing through all the wallets' cards, heading down yesterday's hall to teenage girls writhing, screaming, alone in labor; the baby's breech and we can't turn it around. We can't turn any of it around, doctors yelling (louder than the girl/her Mother) *Jesus Christ*, a name I've heard thousands, maybe millions of times. A name that has no body, but clearly a presence in this land of the sick and troubled. Near its bed or commode or atop an IV pole, I have heard the body's thud. And it's not the tree's apple. The bruising's not the same, for the apple's sob is silence. Not so with the body, for we want a hand up, we want the world to know we've collapsed and the floor's not fit for a bed. The body knows all of this and its voice sings the sounds of hurt and suffering, heaven's black pots and pans thunder down and down. It's the endless choir of cawing crows in a Kansas field, a great dance of fire sweeping a Sequoia forest. You can not forget tears from this smoke, how your face winced against such heat, moving light and heavy trunks, sheets covering the newly fallen. *Because they are you. They are you.* Because even alone, knowing almost no hope, the body will cry, it will cry out until the perfumed bottle of its voice is spent, until the candle's whisper dissolves. And then, urine and feces will hold hands, school children, they'll dance together in one puddle. Because we are all the renters' kids, without shoes or boots, we spray paint X's on blistered walls, the when and where and how we lived until we could no longer stand.

Retired Nurse:
Poetry Reading With My Patients

We are moving from the gymnasium to the football stadium, a voice
calls out to the gathering crowd. Late afternoon, the elders
have a one-day pass, the others, their jobs, children, dreams.
Remember 1976? Being pushed onto Med-Surg wards moss green,
trembling in our new *Clinics*, **Do not expose your patients!**
the mandate ringing in our ears.

Oh, they are bringing my water to the podium, testing the mike.
I'm worried, just a little, that I've not enough books, never sure
If I should bake a cake or buy a pack of Ho Hos. Maybe Amazon
could fly over, drop a crate of *Breathless* or *Tenderly Lift Me*.
Then I remember, I don't really know anybody at Amazon. And
Borders, Barnes and Noble won't carry my small press books.

As I am ushered to the front row, families stand, wave, blow kisses.
I can't believe the banners: Best Enema I Ever Had, My Baby's
IV With One Stick, I Heard You Pray, Dad *Did* Need Surgery,
The Heart Stents Worked, I Stopped Cutting, It *Was* My Gall Bladder,
You Found My Tampon, Sorry For Saying *Fuck*,
My Harley Shirt and Shoulder Mended, Who Be Florence?

I should mention I will be introduced by Emily Dickinson,
Poet Laureate of Heaven (eventually things do get righted),
followed by a brief prayer, an Indiana minister, who at
seventeen walked to my triage desk, complaining neck pain
(a C3 fracture, non-displaced). I assisted with the halo brace,
whispered in his ear *Do something special with your life.*

I can only wonder what it was like for him to walk around
high school looking like Frankenstein for six months. Mom
having to help him bathe. All the questions I might want to ask,
but these black butterflies I've pinned to the page are aching
to fly. Thirty-four years, laying on of hands, lifting
bruised bodies, I can tell you *I didn't sketch nearly enough.*

To paint pastels you must touch faces like Ingrid's,
ninety-two years old, Jewish, her numbers, a blue bracelet on her wrist,
violet eyes a meadow of forgiveness. One student morning,
I took her apical, brushed and wound her white hair's bun.
All that passed between us became a locket on a fine gold chain.
Do something special with your life, her bracelet said.

o

Acknowledgments (continued)

My gratitude to these friends and mentors for their support, critique and fellowship: Maggie Anderson, Alice Cone, Diane Gilliam, Nancy Henderson, Sue Johnson, Katherine Orr, Nicole Pearce and Vivian Pemberton.

Warmest thanks to Michael Shay of the Wyoming Arts Council for the opportunity to juror the 2010 Blanchard/Doubleday fellowship awards.

Continued appreciation to Robert Wick and Walter Wick for providing Kent State University's Stan and Tom Wick Poetry Program.

I thank Mr. Jack Stadler for providing Bucknell University with the Younger Poets Fellowship program.

For the gift of funds and time, I thank the Ohio Arts Council and the Vermont Studio Center. For support and friendship I thank Carol Donley and Martin Kohn, co-founders of the Center for Literature and Medicine at Hiram College.

Love and gratitude to my brothers and sisters of UNA Council 8, AFSCME 2026, Trumbull Memorial Hospital, Warren, Ohio. I especially thank ICU nurses Donna Fickes, Cheri Pennock and Mary Jo Bofenkamp. For supporting early writing endeavors, I thank Elizabeth Hoobler, Gloria Young, Sandy Marovitz, Gary Ciuba, Mary Ann Lowry, Mary Turzillo, Susanna Fein, Robin Becker, Brigit Kelly, and Colette Inez.

Forever, all love to my family, especially David for his good heart/ keen eyes and my grandson, Tony for his phone calls.

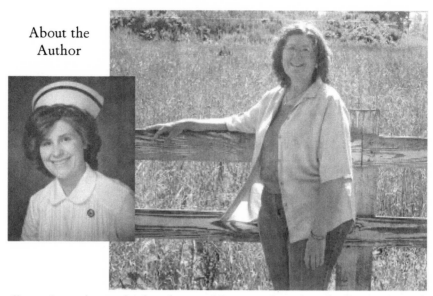

About the
Author

(Jeanne's nursing graduation photo and Jeanne today; photo by Tammy Streets)

Jeanne Bryner was born in Appalachia and grew up in Newton Falls, Ohio. She is a practicing registered nurse and a graduate of Trumbull Memorial Hospital's School of Nursing and Kent State University's Honors College. Her books include *Breathless, Blind Horse: Poems, Eclipse: Stories, Tenderly Lift Me: Nurses Honored, Celebrated and Remembered, The Wedding of Miss Meredith Mouse* and *No Matter How Many Windows,* the story of women in her family which won the 2011 Tillie Olsen Award for Creative Writing from the Working Class Studies Association. Her poetry has been adapted for the stage and performed in Ohio, New York, Texas, Kentucky, West Virginia, California and Edinburgh, Scotland. Her new play, *Foxglove Canyon,* was first performed in Akron for Summa Healthcare's Humanities' conference under the direction of Russell Zampino. With the support of Hiram College's Center for Literature, Medicine and Biomedical Humanities, her nursing poetry has been adapted for the stage and performed by Verb Ballets, Cleveland, Ohio. As a community affiliate of Youngstown State University's Center for Working Class Studies, she frequently treats working-class issues. She teaches writing workshops in schools, universities, community centers, cancer support groups and assisted living facilities. She has received writing fellowships from Bucknell University, the Ohio Arts Council (1997, 2007), and Vermont Studio Center. She lives with her husband in Newton Falls, Ohio.

About the Artist

Judy Waid is retired after forty years of nursing. A graduate of Trumbull Memorial Hospital's School of Nursing, wife and mother, she has always pursued her love of art. She studied at Kent State University and the Cleveland Institute of Art and has received several art awards. The Ohio Nurses Association commissioned her to design medallions based on nursing personalities and historical moments in nursing now in museums, universities, private collections, and in the textbook *Nursing, The Finest Art*. Her portraits of prominent women in the Warren-Youngstown area are well known and on display at the Warren Trumbull County Public Library and the Harriet Upton House. A member of the Trumbull Art Gallery and its portrait group, she lives with her husband in Howland, Ohio.

RECENT BOOKS BY
BOTTOM DOG PRESS

Working Lives Series

Smoke: Poems by Jeanne Bryner 96 pgs. $16

Maggot : A Novel by Robert Flanaga, 262 pgs. $18

Broken Collar: A Novel by Ron Mitchell, 234 pgs. $18

The Pattern Maker's Daughter: Poems
by Sandee Gertz Umbach, 90 pages $16

The Way-Back Room: Memoir of a Detroit Childhood
by Mary Minock, 216 pgs. $18

The Free Farm: A Novel by Larry Smith, 306 pgs. $18

Sinners of Sanction County: Stories
by Charles Dodd White, 160 pgs. $17

Learning How: Stories, Yarns & Tales
by Richard Hague, 216 pgs. $18

Strangers in America: A Novel
by Erika Meyers, 140 pgs. $16

Riders on the Storm: A Novel
by Susan Streeter Carpenter, 404 pgs. $18

The Long River Home
by Larry Smith, 230 pgs. cloth $22; paper $16

Landscape with Fragmented Figures
by Jeff Vande Zande, 232 pgs. $16

The Big Book of Daniel: Collected Poems
by Daniel Thompson, 340 pgs. cloth $22; paper $18

Reply to an Eviction Notice: Poems
by Robert Flanagan, 100 pgs. $15

An Unmistakable Shade of Red & The Obama Chronicles
by Mary E. Weems, 80 pgs. $15

d.a.levy & the mimeograph revolution
eds. Ingrid Swanberg & Larry Smith, 276 pgs. & dvd $25

Our Way of Life: Poems by Ray McNiece, 128 pgs. $15

http://smithdocs.net

CPSIA information can be obtained at www.ICGtesting.com
Printed in the USA
BVOW042024010712

294048BV00001B/56/P